METABOLISM BOOSTING

SMOOTHIES AND JUICES

Over 75 Fresh and Healthy Recipes

Tina Haupert

CIDER MILL
PRESS

BOOK
PUBLISHERS

Kennebunkport, Maine

13-Digit ISBN: 978-1-60433-539-2
10-Digit ISBN: 1-60433-539-4

This book may be ordered by mail from the publisher. Please include $4.95 for postage and handling. Please support your local bookseller first!

Books published by Cider Mill Press Book Publishers are available at special discounts for bulk purchases in the United States by corporations, institutions, and other organizations. For more information, please contact the publisher.

Cider Mill Press Book Publishers
"Where good books are ready for press"
12 Spring Street
PO Box 454
Kennebunkport, Maine 04046

Visit us on the Web!
www.cidermillpress.com

Design by Emily Regis
Typography: Gill Sans, MrsEaves, and Avenir
All images used under license from Shutterstock.com.
Printed in China

1 2 3 4 5 6 7 8 9 0
First Edition

TABLE *of* CONTENTS

READY TO REV YOUR METABOLISM?

Metabolism is a group of complex body processes that in part make up a person's basal metabolic rate or the rate of burning calories at a standstill. Everyone wanting to lose weight wants their metabolic rate (or metabolism) to be higher. Certain foods and beverages are known to have particular nutrients that provide a metabolism boost. Protein utilizes more calories to process than the ingestion of carbohydrates and fats. Spicy foods and caffeine provide a temporary boost to your metabolism. Certain foods high in specific minerals such as iron and selenium help support thyroid function, which can improve our basal metabolic rate. There is also research to support that foods low in sugar and high in fiber (like non-starchy vegetables) and healthy fats help reduce insulin levels, which cause the body to utilize food more efficiently and prevent it from storing it as body fat.

Both juices and smoothies provide lots of nutrients that may help you lose weight. But they differ in the effect they have on blood sugar. Smoothies blend whole foods (such as fruits and vegetables) that contain fiber that the body does not digest. This helps to keep you fuller for longer and maintain lower blood sugar levels. Juices provide little to no fiber but because they are more concentrated can provide more nutrients (vitamins, minerals, and phytonutrients) per serving.

Juices and smoothies are easy and tasty ways to get more healthy superfoods in your diet. Find what you enjoy, and don't be afraid to be a little creative and experiment.

The Skinny on Metabolism–Boosting Foods

We've got plenty of tasty recipes for juices and smoothies with metabolism-boosting ingredients. Once you get used to juicing and making smoothies, you'll quickly start getting creative and making your own combinations. Here are some metabolism-boosting ingredients.

High-iron foods: Spinach, kale, parsley, dandelion greens, chili peppers, sesame seeds, pumpkin seeds, beet greens, collard greens, romaine lettuce.

Selenium-rich foods: Brazil nuts, spinach, sunflower seeds, broccoli, Swiss chard.

Omega-3 foods: Chia sees, hemp seeds, flaxseeds, walnuts, almonds, almond butter.

High-protein foods: Whey protein, rice protein, hemp protein, Greek-style unsweetened yogurt.

High-caffeine foods: Dark chocolate, coffee, green tea.

Herbs and spices: Cinnamon.

Spicy foods: Chili peppers.

Practical Tips

Because juicing machines and fresh produce vary so much and will give you different results, the juice recipes in this book produce one serving, which is equal to approximately 8 ounces of liquid.

Wash and (if necessary) cut all fruits and vegetables before putting them into the blender or juicer. Remove any bruised or damaged parts. When you can, choose fresh, ripe, organic produce.

Remove pits and seeds from fruit before juicing to prevent damaging machine parts. To help prevent pulp from clogging the machine, alternate soft/wet and hard/leafy produce whenever possible.

Do not pour water, coconut water, or other juices directly into juicer unless specifically directed to do so.

Our smoothie recipes call for whey protein, but you can also use casein or egg white or any of the vegan protein powders on the market (including soy, pea, hemp, or rice).

— Breea Johnson, M.S., R.D., L.D.N.

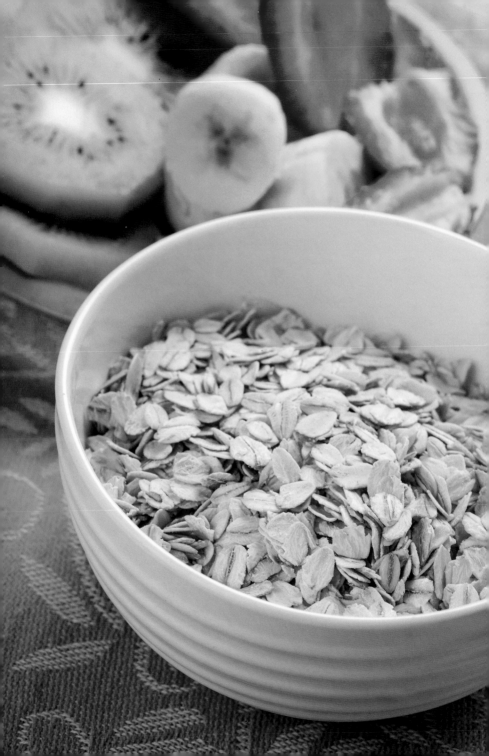

BREAKFAST SMOOTHIES

Rise and shine! We all know breakfast is the most important meal of the day, so you want to make sure it's both nutritious and satisfying. Plus, eating a healthy breakfast sets the tone for your morning, which can help you make smart choices all day long. For these reasons, smoothies are the perfect choice for a quick, nutritious, and delicious breakfast.

The smoothies in this chapter are packed with flavor and nutrients and guaranteed to keep your belly full and happy all morning long. For some added satiety, try a scoop of protein powder in any of these recipes. The protein powder will likely thicken the smoothie, so be ready to add a splash of additional liquid to get it to your preferred consistency.

If you're typically rushed in the morning, you can make these smoothies ahead of time. Either add all the ingredients to your blender the night before and refrigerate it overnight to make in the morning, or blend your breakfast smoothie, store it in a travel-friendly container, and then just give it a quick shake in the morning.

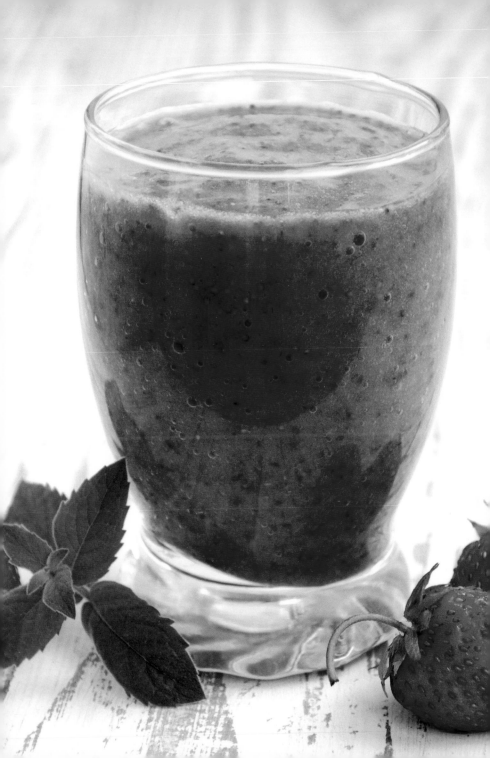

STRAWBERRY-POMEGRANATE SMOOTHIE

Strawberries and pomegranate combine in this intensely sweet and fresh smoothie. Banana adds a wonderfully thick, creaminess without overpowering the other flavors. This smoothie might just be one of your favorites!

 ½ banana

 1 cup frozen strawberries

 1 cup pomegranate juice

Combine ingredients in a blender until smooth. Pour into a glass and enjoy immediately.

Bonus Recipe

BERRY BEE
For extra sweetness, add 2 tbsp honey (or agave nectar, if you're on a vegan diet).

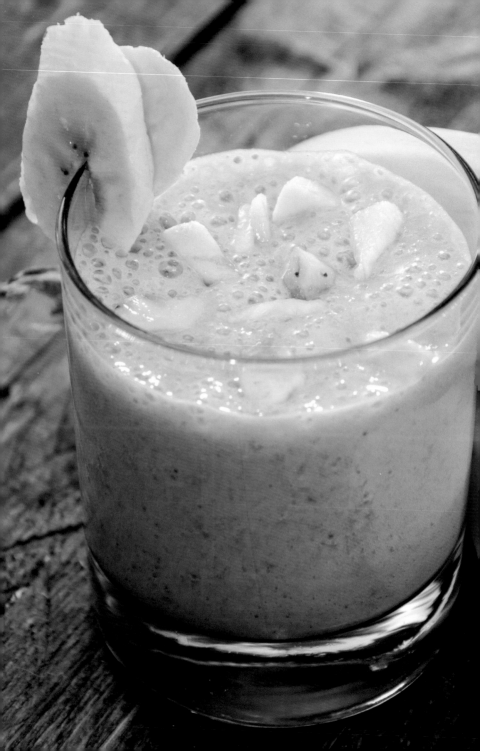

BANANA BREAD SMOOTHIE

This smoothie will remind you of banana bread for breakfast.
Bonus: It's faster and healthier.

---

 1 frozen banana

 ¼ cup rolled oats

 1 cup almond milk

 1 scoop (20g) vanilla whey powder

 1 tbsp ground flaxseed meal

 1 tbsp honey (or agave nectar)

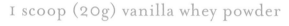 2 tbsp chopped walnuts

Combine ingredients in a blender until smooth. Pour into a glass and enjoy immediately.

Bonus Recipe

 ## BANANA BREAD & MILK SMOOTHIE
Replace the almond milk and whey powder with fat-free milk and low-fat yogurt.

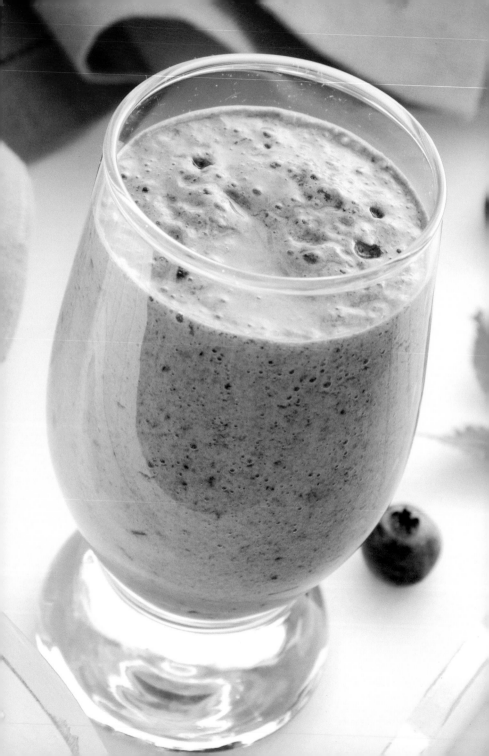

PEANUT BUTTER & JELLY SMOOTHIE

Just about everyone likes peanut butter and jelly sandwiches:
They're a quick and easy meal that fills you up and tastes great—
and same goes with this smoothie!

 1 cup frozen blueberries

 1½ cups almond milk

 2–3 tbsp peanut butter

 1 tbsp honey (or agave nectar)

 ¼ tsp vanilla extract

4–5 ice cubes

Combine ingredients in a blender until smooth. Pour into a glass and enjoy immediately.

Bonus Recipe

PB & BLACKBERRY JAM SMOOTHIE

 Replace the frozen blueberries with frozen raspberries.

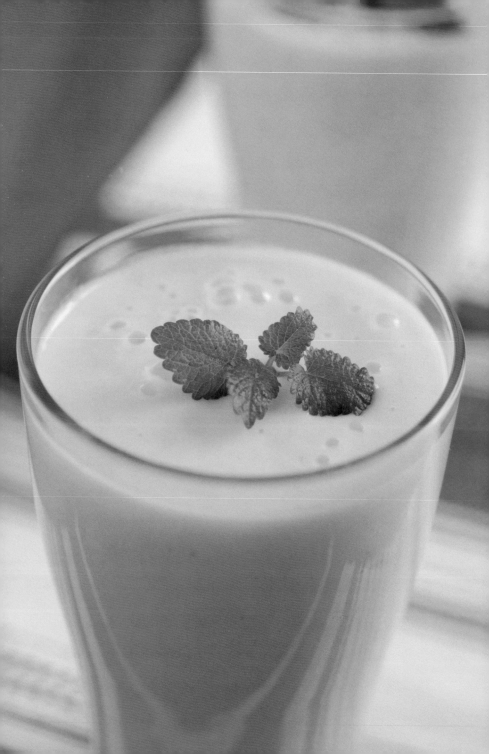

MIGHTY MANGO SMOOTHIE

This Mighty Mango Smoothie will get you moving in the morning. Bold mango and pineapple flavors awaken your senses, and whey powder keeps your stomach satisfied all morning long.

---

1 cup frozen mango chunks

½ cup frozen pineapple chunks

1 scoop (20 g) vanilla whey powder

1 cup almond milk

¾ cup coconut water

Combine ingredients in a blender until smooth. Pour into a glass and enjoy immediately.

Bonus Recipe

TROPICAL PINEAPPLE SMOOTHIE
Instead of mango, use 1 ½ cups of chunked frozen pineapple for an extra tropical-tasting smoothie.

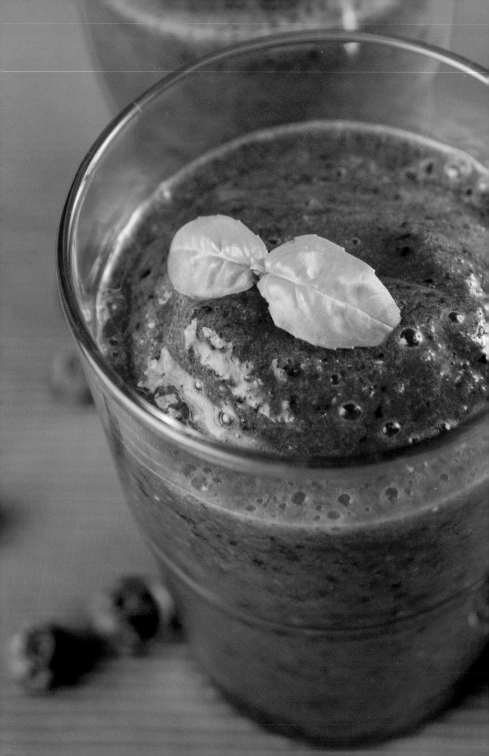

BLUEBERRY-BASIL SMOOTHIE

From your first sip of this smoothie, the flavors of blueberries, basil, and lemon will give you a natural lift to get you going.

 ½ cup blueberries

 ½ frozen banana

 1 handful of spinach

 1½ cups almond milk

 1 tbsp freshly squeezed lemon juice *optional*

 A small handful of fresh basil leaves (approximately 10–12)

Combine ingredients in a blender until smooth. Pour into a glass and enjoy immediately.

Bonus Recipe

BLUEBERRY-MINT SMOOTHIE
For a minty-fresh smoothie, swap out the basil for 8–10 fresh mint leaves before blending.

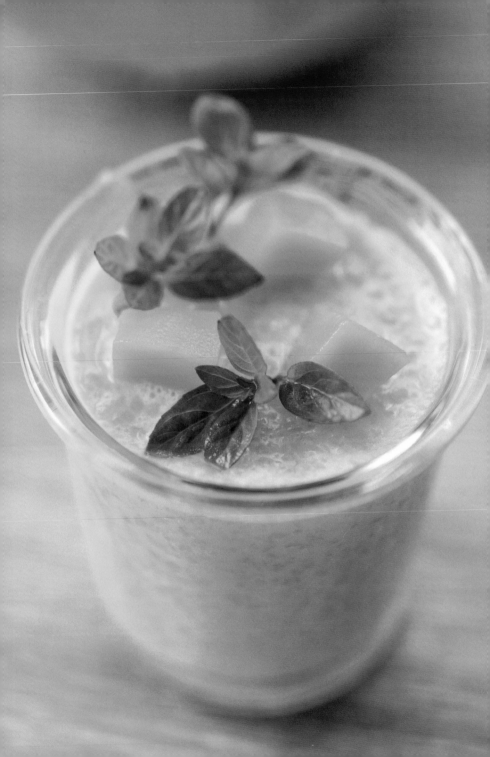

ORANGE ENERGIZER SMOOTHIE

This bright-orange smoothie will get your attention in more ways than one. Pineapple, pumpkin, orange juice, and freshly grated ginger pack a serious flavor punch.

 ½ cup frozen pineapple chunks

 ½ cup pumpkin puree

 ½ cup Greek-style yogurt

 ¾ cup orange juice

 1 tbsp maple syrup

 ½ tsp cinnamon

 2 tsp freshly grated ginger

 8–10 fresh mint leaves *optional*

4–5 ice cubes

Combine ingredients in a blender until smooth. Pour into a glass, garnish with mint leaves if you'd like, and enjoy immediately.

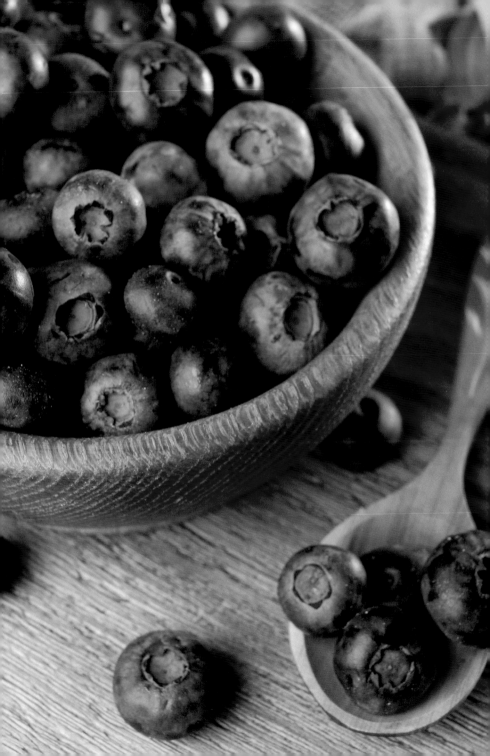

WORKOUT SMOOTHIES

When it comes to fitness, if you've started to notice that your muscles don't recover as quickly as they used to and your performance is more sluggish than in the past, try focusing more on good post-workout nutrition. The key to proper recovery is consuming 10–20 grams of protein within 30 minutes of completing your workout. Drinking smoothies is a convenient way to get these essential nutrients in your diet.

The smoothies in this chapter include nutritious ingredients that help fight inflammation and promote quick repair and healing inside the body, which is especially important for overcoming soreness and getting you out the door for your next workout. All these recipes include nutritional powerhouse ingredients. From bananas and cherries to coconut water and chia seeds—you'll get the nutrients you need for recovery.

These smoothies call for whey powder. If you follow a vegan diet, there are several vegan protein powders available, including those made from soy, peas, hemp, and rice.

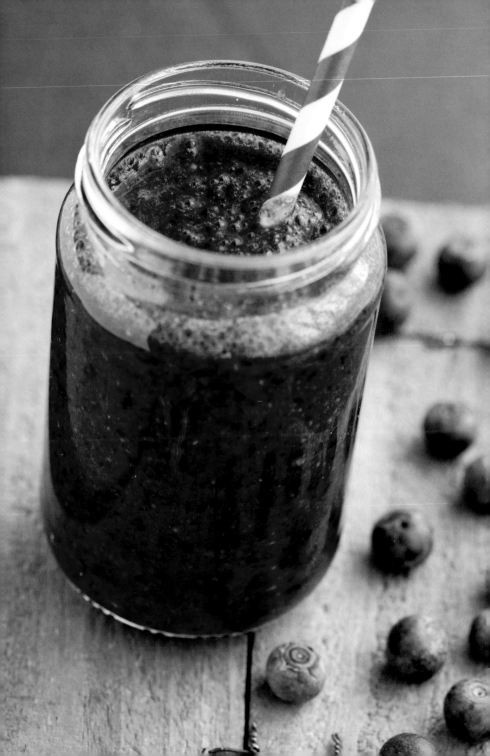

ULTIMATE RECOVERY SMOOTHIE

This smoothie has an all-star cast of ingredients that are essential to proper recovery after a workout.

 ½ cup frozen cherries

 ½ cup frozen blueberries

 ½ cup chopped spinach

 ½ cup almond milk

 ½ cup coconut water

 1 scoop (20g) vanilla whey powder

 2 tsp chia seeds or hemp seeds

Combine ingredients in a blender until smooth. Pour into a glass and enjoy immediately.

Bonus Recipe

STRAWBERRY RECOVERY SMOOTHIE
Swap out blueberries for ½ cup frozen strawberries.

CREAMY CHOCOLATE PROTEIN SMOOTHIE

Tough workout? If so, you might be looking for a sweet reward for all of your hard work. This smoothie provides protein to your muscles for quick recovery while tasting like a delectable chocolate dessert at the same time!

---

 1 frozen banana

 ½ cup frozen chopped spinach

 ½ avocado, peeled and pitted

 1¼ cups chocolate almond milk

 1 scoop (20g) chocolate whey powder

 2 tsp chia seeds *optional*

Combine ingredients in a blender until smooth. Pour into a glass and enjoy immediately.

NUT BUTTER AND BANANA SMOOTHIE

This peanut butter and banana smoothie is loaded with protein to help you recover after your workout and keep you satisfied.

 1 frozen banana

 2 heaping tbsp of almond or peanut butter

 1¼ cups vanilla almond milk

 1 scoop (20g) vanilla whey powder

 ½ tsp vanilla extract

 ¼ tsp cinnamon

Combine ingredients in a blender until smooth. Pour into a glass and enjoy immediately.

Bonus Recipe

 ## CHOCOLATE NUT SMOOTHIE
Replace the vanilla almond milk with chocolate almond milk and the vanilla whey powder with chocolate whey powder.

SQUASH SORENESS SMOOTHIE

The variety of nutrients in this smoothie promote quick repair and healing after a workout, which is important for overcoming soreness and getting you out the door for your next sweat session.

 ½ banana

 ½ cup frozen pineapple chunks

 ½ cup frozen diced butternut squash

 I scoop (20g) vanilla whey powder

 I cup coconut water

 2 tsp honey (or agave nectar)

 I tsp chia seeds

 ¼ tsp cinnamon

Combine ingredients in a blender until smooth. Pour into a glass and enjoy immediately.

VANILLA NUT SMOOTHIE

Sweet, nutty, and, oh, so delicious! Every time I make this smoothie, I slug it down in a matter of minutes, which is important for refueling muscles with essential vitamins and minerals immediately after exercise.

---

 1 frozen banana

 2 tbsp almond butter

 1¼ cups vanilla almond milk

 1 scoop (20g) vanilla whey powder

 1 tbsp ground flaxseed meal

 1 tbsp honey

Combine ingredients in a blender until smooth. Pour into a glass and enjoy immediately.

Bonus Recipe

VANILLA-MAPLE NUT SMOOTHIE
Replace the honey with a tablespoon or two of maple syrup.

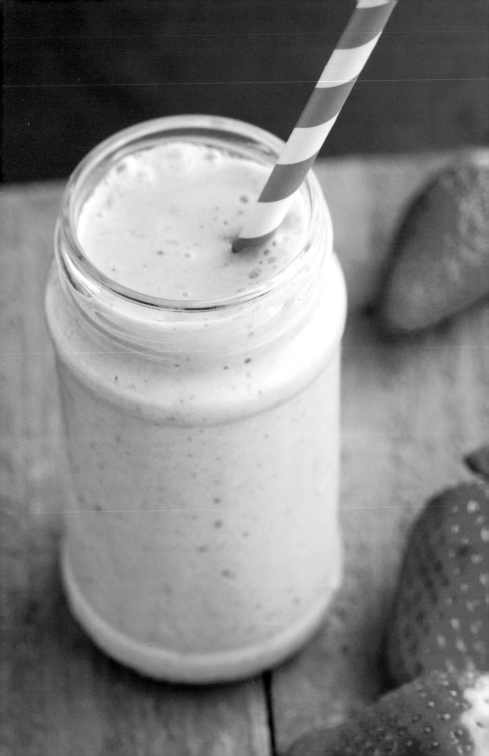

STRAWBERRY-ALMOND SMOOTHIE

Strawberries and almonds come together in this dessert-like smoothie. You might think the taste is too good to be true, but it's actually a wonderful recovery smoothie too, thanks to all of the muscle-repairing nutrients.

 I cup frozen strawberries

 2 tbsp almond butter

 1½ cups vanilla almond milk

1 scoop (20g) vanilla whey powder

2 tbsp sliced almonds *optional*

Combine ingredients in a blender until smooth. Pour into a glass and enjoy immediately.

Bonus Recipe

BANANA SPLIT SMOOTHIE
Replace the vanilla whey powder with chocolate whey powder, add a frozen banana, and skip the sliced almonds.

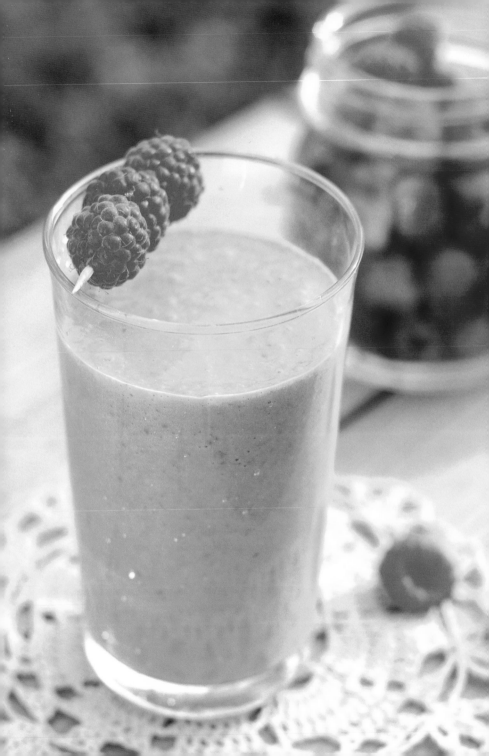

COCO-CHOCO-RASPBERRY SMOOTHIE

Rehydrate and replenish with this delicious smoothie made with raspberries, coconut, and protein powder.

---

 1 cup frozen raspberries

 1 cup coconut milk

 ¼ cup coconut water

 1 scoop (20g) chocolate whey powder

 2 tbsp shredded coconut

Combine ingredients in a blender until smooth. Pour into a glass and enjoy immediately.

Bonus Recipe

COCO POWER BURST
Add 2 cups baby spinach.

Coconut water is rich in electrolytes and potassium, which makes it great for rehydration after exercise.

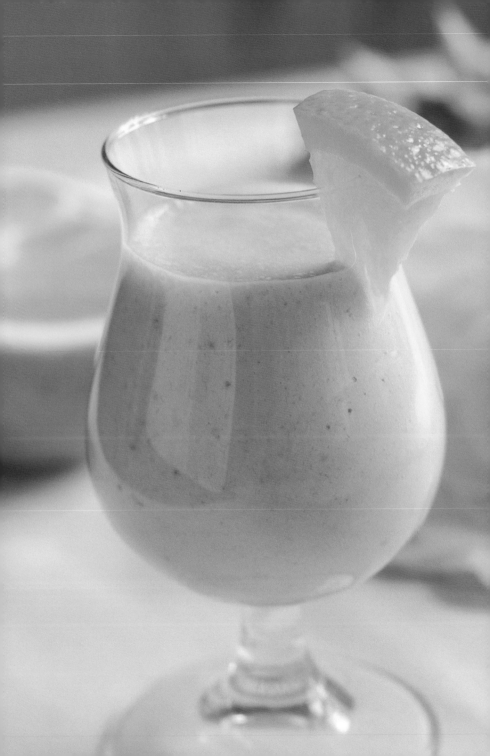

ORANGE CREAMSICLE SMOOTHIE

You finished a tough workout! Congrats!

 I cup orange juice

 6–8 ounces vanilla-flavored yogurt

 ½ frozen banana

 I scoop (20g) vanilla whey powder

 2 tsp honey (or agave nectar) *optional*

4–5 ice cubes

Combine ingredients in a blender until smooth. Pour into a glass and enjoy immediately.

Bonus Recipe

 ## COLADA CREAMSICLE
Replace the banana with ½ cup fresh or frozen pineapple and add 2 tbsp shredded coconut.

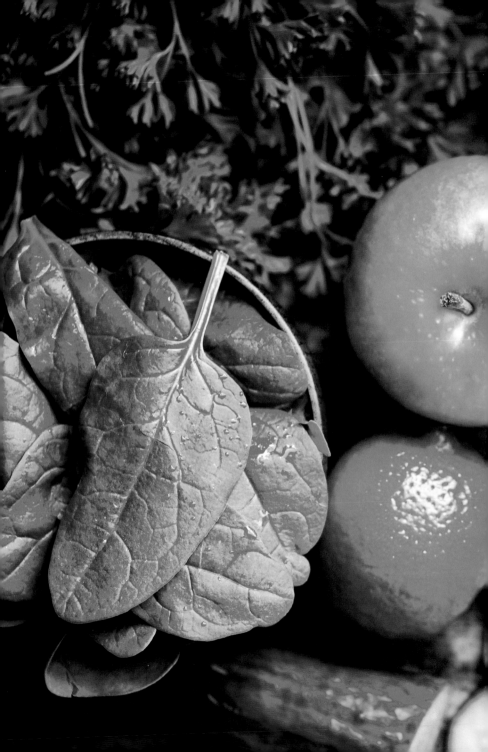

GREEN SMOOTHIES AND JUICES

The recipes in this chapter have one obvious thing in common: They're green. Less obvious is how truly nutritious they are for you. Leafy greens—the darker the better—are a rich source of minerals, including iron, calcium, potassium, and magnesium, as well as vitamins K, C, E, and many of the B vitamins. In addition, they provide a variety of phytonutrients and even small amounts of omega-3 fats. With such a wealth of health in a glass, it's no wonder the green juice trend has caught on. It's an incredibly healthy way to boost your vitality and wellness.

Vegetables in a smoothie? It might sound a bit odd and perhaps not very appetizing. But you'll be surprised how delicious a green smoothie can be. Many of us don't typically eat raw spinach or parsley on a regular basis— at least not in the amount called for in a green smoothie. But when these leafy greens are blended with sweet fruits, such as bananas, the flavor is transformed. And if spicy is more your thing, we've got a Spicy Green Smoothie to get your metabolism—and taste buds—jumping!

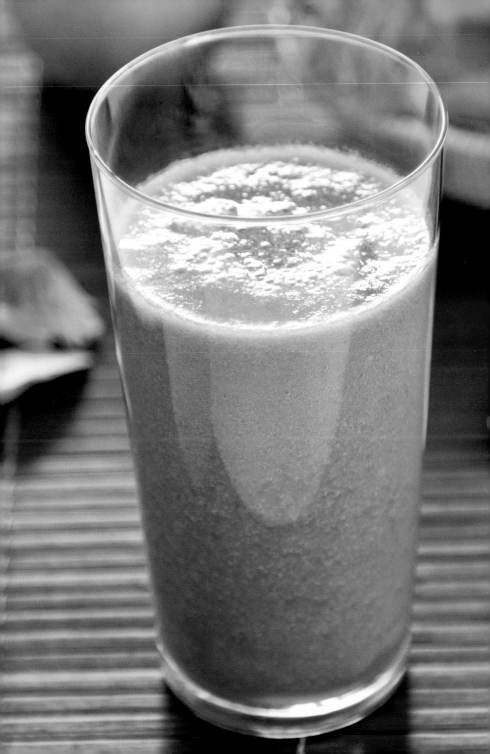

EVERYDAY GREEN JUICE

This is my go-to green juice recipe. Besides being delicious, it also has a great mix of flavors and nutrients. I always feel healthier after I drink a glass of this Everyday Green Juice.

---

 4 ounces of fresh spinach or kale

 1 apple

 1 cucumber

 4 celery stalks

 Fresh ginger root to taste *optional*

Put ingredients into a juicer, alternating greens with chunked fruits and veggies. Pour into a glass or over ice and drink immediately.

Bonus Recipe

GREEN CITRUS SMOOTHIE

 For a citrusy kick, add the juice of a quarter or half of a lemon or lime.

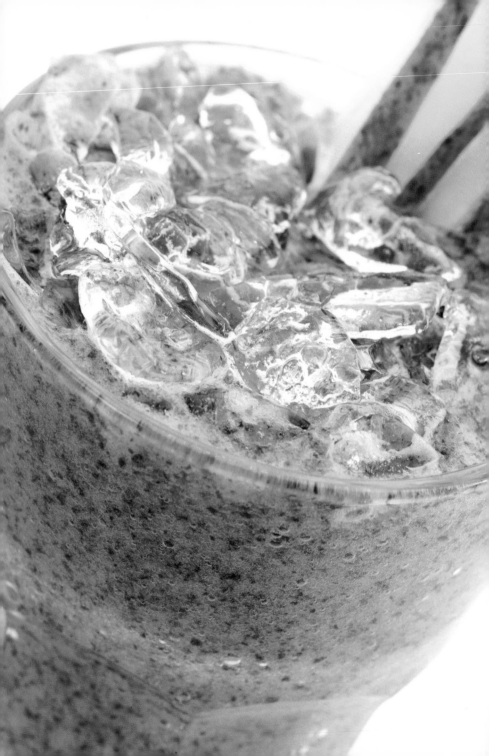

SPINACH-PEAR JUICE

Simple and nutritious, this juice comes together in matter of minutes, thanks to just three ingredients.

 3 pears

 2–4 ounces spinach

 ½ cucumber

Put ingredients into a juicer, alternating greens with chunked fruits and veggies. Pour into a glass and drink immediately.

Bonus Recipe

PERFECT PEAR JUICE
Replace the cucumber with a Granny Smith apple.

Pears are a good source of vitamin C! A medium-sized pear contains about 10 percent of your daily recommended value. In addition, pears are loaded with phytonutrients and antioxidants, a variety of which are found in the vibrantly colored skins.

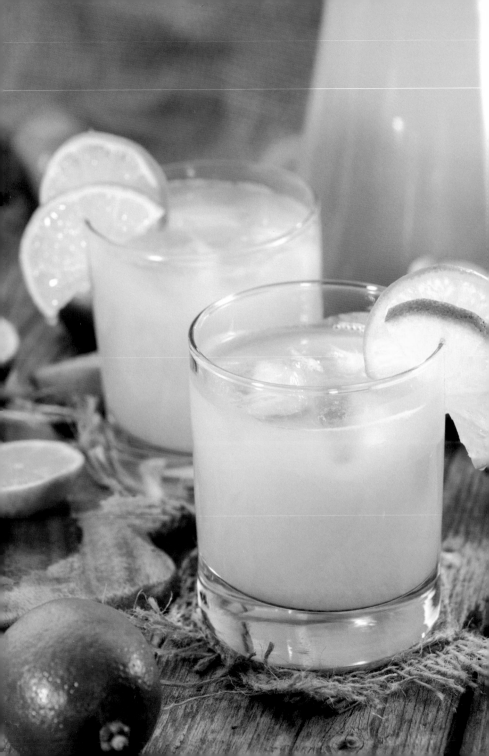

MINT-APPLE-LIME JUICE

Sweet, sour, bitter, refreshing… this juice will definitely keep your taste buds guessing!

 2 apples

 1 cucumber

 1 handful of fresh spinach or other leafy green

 ½ lime

 10—12 leaves of fresh mint

Put ingredients into a juicer, alternating greens with chunked fruits and veggies. Pour into a glass or over ice and drink immediately.

Bonus Recipe

MINT-APPLE-LIME REFRESHER

 For a refreshing spritzer, leave out the cucumber and greens, and mix your fresh juice with crushed ice and club soda.

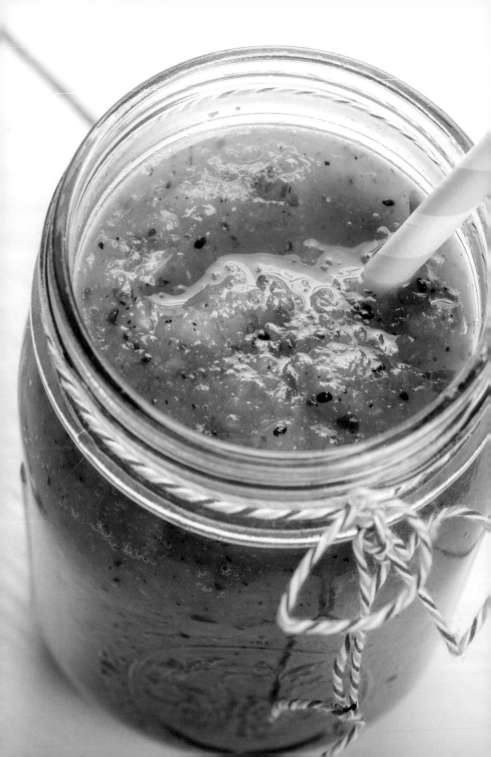

GREEN LEMON-LIME TWIST

The ingredients in this mellow, green juice might seem simple, but you'll be thoroughly impressed by their interesting and refreshing flavors.

 2 ounces dark leafy greens of your choice

 1 apple

 1 lemon

 1 lime

 6 celery stalks

Put ingredients into a juicer, alternating greens with chunked fruits and veggies. Pour into a glass or over ice and drink immediately.

Bonus Recipe

 ## SWEET GREEN TWIST
For a sweeter version, replace the celery stalks with one kiwi, peeled and chopped.

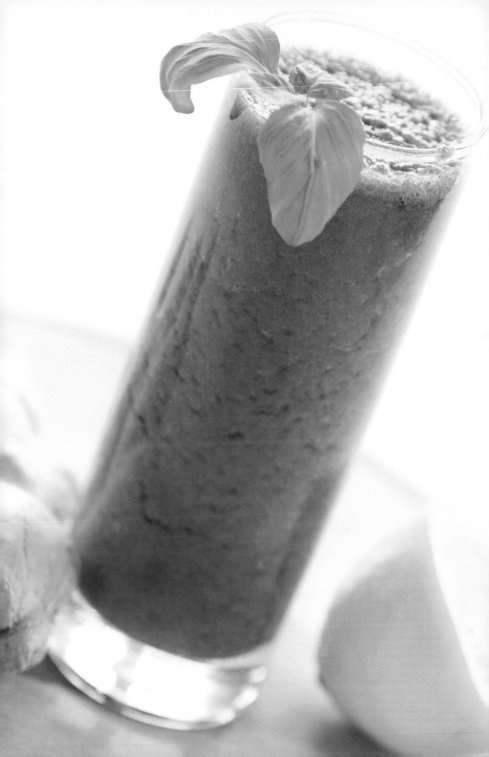

ZESTY GREEN GINGER JUICE

Looking for something to really wake you up? Perhaps something a little zesty? Here's the juice for you! Beware: It's got a little bite.

---

 2 lemons, peeled and sliced

 1 handful of spinach or kale

 4 stalks of celery

 ½ Granny Smith apple

 Fresh ginger root to taste

Put ingredients into a juicer, alternating greens with chunked fruits and veggies. Pour into a glass or over ice and drink immediately.

Bonus Recipe

 ## SWEET GREEN GINGER JUICE
For a sweeter and mellower juice, replace lemons with two apples.

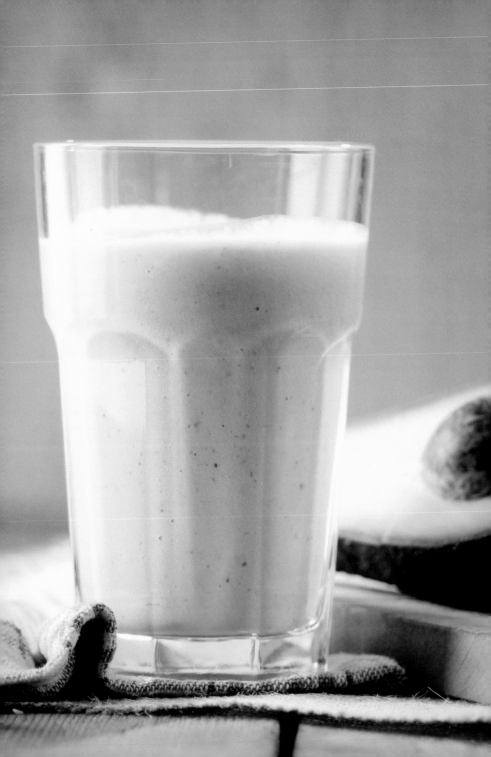

CREAMY AVOCADO SMOOTHIE

Avocado in a smoothie? You bet! It adds a wonderfully creamy texture and a colorful hue. This smoothie will seriously satisfy both your stomach and taste buds.

 1 frozen banana

 ½ cup frozen chopped spinach

 ½ avocado, peeled and pitted

 1¼ cups vanilla almond milk

 1 tbsp honey (or agave nectar)

 ¼ tsp cinnamon

Combine ingredients in a blender until smooth. Pour into a glass and serve immediately.

Bonus Recipe

 ## AVOCADO CREAMSICLE
Replace the spinach and almond milk with ½ cup plain Greek yogurt and ½ cup orange juice.

COCONUT-KALE SMOOTHIE

A taste of the tropics! Loaded with kale, banana, and ground flaxseed, this nutrient-rich smoothie is so delicious and refreshing, you won't even know it's good for you.

---

 1 frozen banana

 1 cup frozen chopped kale

 1 ½ cups coconut milk

 1 tbsp ground flaxseed meal

 1 tbsp honey (or agave nectar)

 ¼ tsp coconut extract

Combine ingredients in a blender until smooth. Pour into a glass and serve immediately.

SPICY GREEN SMOOTHIE

Ready for a little spice? This smoothie combines jalapeño and cayenne pepper for an exciting flavor. Drink this smoothie when you want a little zip in your life!

 1 large handful of spinach

 ½ cucumber, cut into pieces

 2 celery stalks

 1 lemon, peeled

 1 cup water

 ½ bunch of flat-leaf parsley

 ½ jalapeño, seeded

 ¼ tsp cayenne pepper

 Pinch of sea salt

Combine ingredients in a blender until smooth. Pour into a glass and enjoy immediately.

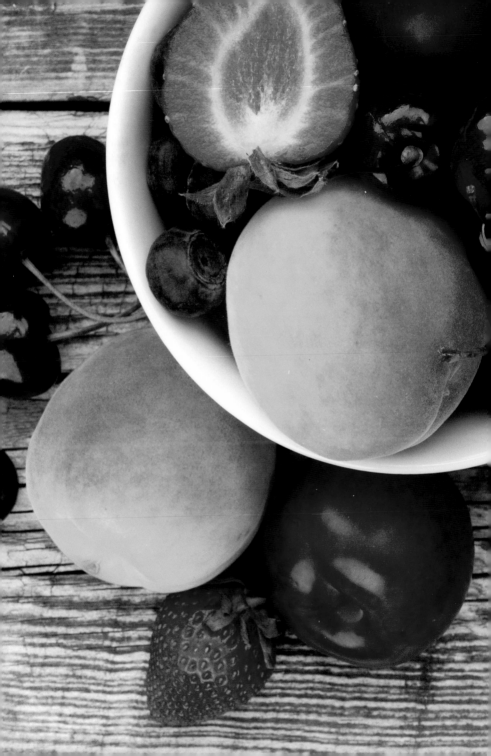

FRUIT JUICE BLENDS

Fruit juice is a wonderful way to add nutrients to your diet. But most store-bought varieties aren't made with 100% juice and are laden with sugar or artificial sweeteners. You can do better at home!

Making freshly pressed fruit juice is a great way to add nutrients to your diet, especially if you sneak in a few vegetables—like carrots—while you're at it. If you're not a big veggie eater, fruit juice blends make it easy to consume them—oftentimes without even tasting them.

These juice blends are high in vitamin C, which—as we all know—is essential to a strong immune system.

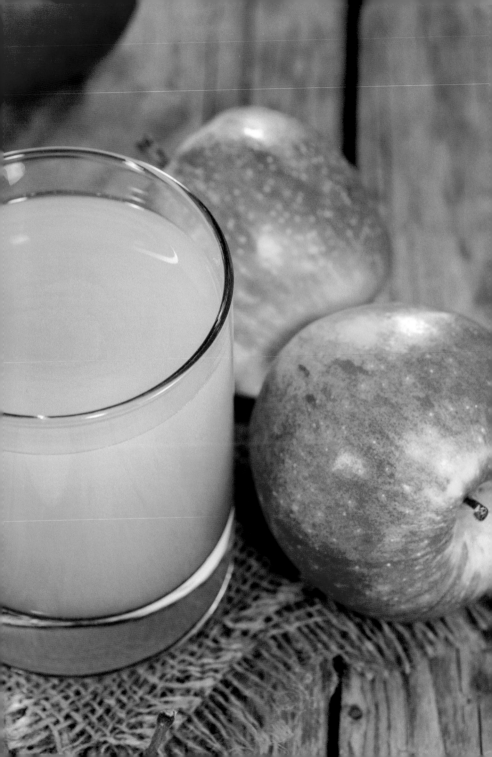

CRISP APPLE JUICE

Imagine biting into a fresh, right-off-the-tree apple. This juice blend tastes just like that—crisp and delicious!

---

 2 apples

 1 cup green grapes

 ¼ lemon, peeled and segmented

Combine all ingredients in a juicer. Pour juice into a glass or over ice and drink immediately.

Bonus Recipe

APPLE "TART"

 Replace one of the apples with ½ lime, peeled and segmented.

You've heard the old saying "an apple a day keeps the doctor away." Because of their high vitamin C content, frequently using apples in your smoothies may indeed help your body fight off colds and other illnesses.

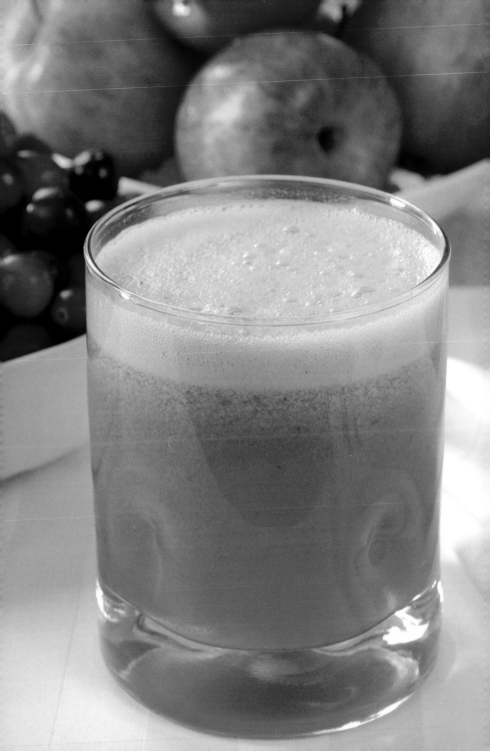

CRAN-APPLE-ORANGE JUICE

Tart cranberries combine with sweet apple and orange for a tangy juice blend that you will love. Cranberries are a good source of vitamin C, E, and fiber as well as dental health.

---

 2 apples

 1 orange, peeled and segmented

 1 cup cranberries

Combine all ingredients in a juicer. Pour juice into a glass or over ice and drink immediately.

Bonus Recipe

CRAN-APPLE-BERRY JUICE
Instead of an orange, substitute 1 cup of fresh strawberries.

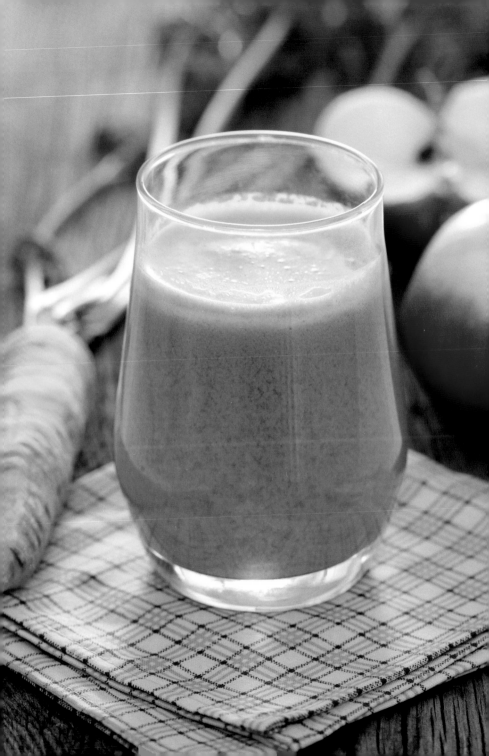

PINEAPPLE-GINGER-CARROT JUICE

This unique blend of tangy and sweet citrus juice packs a punch with a healthy dose of fresh ginger. You're guaranteed a refreshing taste experience.

 ½ apple

 1 cup of fresh pineapple, cut into chunks

 4 carrots

 Fresh ginger root to taste

Combine all ingredients in a juicer. Pour juice into a glass or over ice and drink immediately.

Bonus Recipe

COOL CARROT JUICE
Instead of the apple, use ½ cucumber.

Ginger is loaded with phytonutrients, which may help protect again a variety of diseases, including cancer and heart disease.

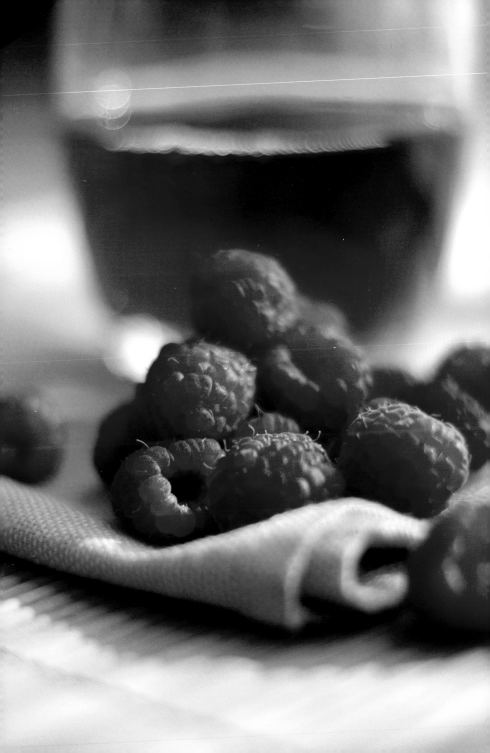

BERRY BLEND

Here's a sweet berry blend for you! Pick your choice of fresh berries and then juice them with cantaloupe and red or green grapes. You're definitely in for a treat!

---

 2 cups fresh mixed berries
blueberries, blackberries, or raspberries

 1 cup cantaloupe, cut into chunks

 ½ cup green or red grapes

Combine all ingredients in a juicer. Pour juice into a glass or over ice and drink immediately.

Bonus Recipe

 ## BERRY-MELON BLEND
Replace cantaloupe with 1 cup of watermelon.

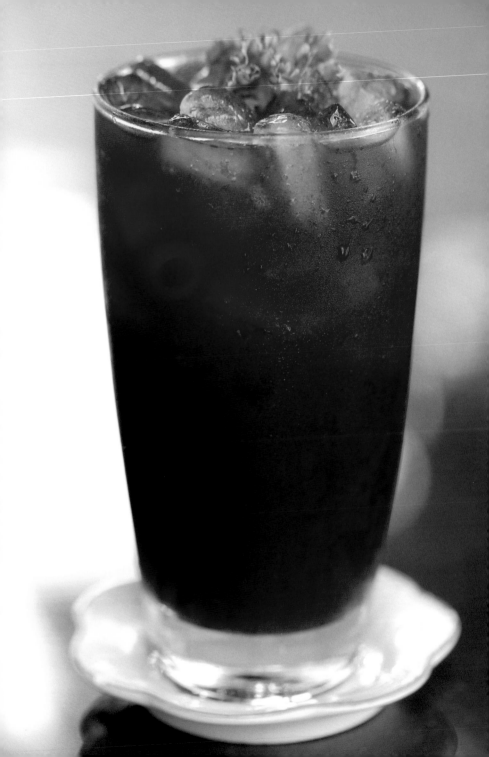

PLUM-BLUEBERRY JUICE

Plums and blueberries—what a delicious combination!

---

 3 plums, pitted

 1 cup blueberries

 1 apple

 ½ cucumber

Combine all ingredients in a juicer. Pour juice into a glass or over ice and drink immediately.

Bonus Recipe

 ## PLUM-APPLE JUICE
Skip the blueberries and cucumber and use three apples instead of one.

Plums are a good source of potassium, a mineral that helps manage high blood pressure and reduces the risk of stroke. In addition, plums contain lutein, an antioxidant that may help promote skin and eye health.

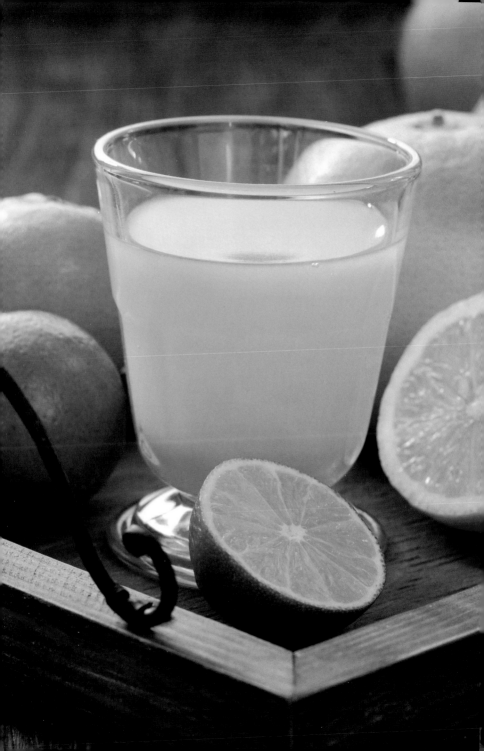

VITAMIN C BLEND

Vitamin C to the rescue! Feeling a little sluggish and need a natural boost? This juice is for you. Loaded with all sorts of vitamin-rich ingredients, this citrus blend tastes great and provides your daily dose of vitamin C.

 2 oranges

 2 kiwis, peeled

 ½ pink grapefruit, peeled and sectioned

 ¼ lime

 ¼ lemon

 Fresh ginger root to taste *optional*

Combine all ingredients in a juicer. Pour juice into a glass or over ice and drink immediately.

Bonus Recipe

 ## THE COLD FIGHTER
After juicing ingredients, add ½ tsp of cinnamon.

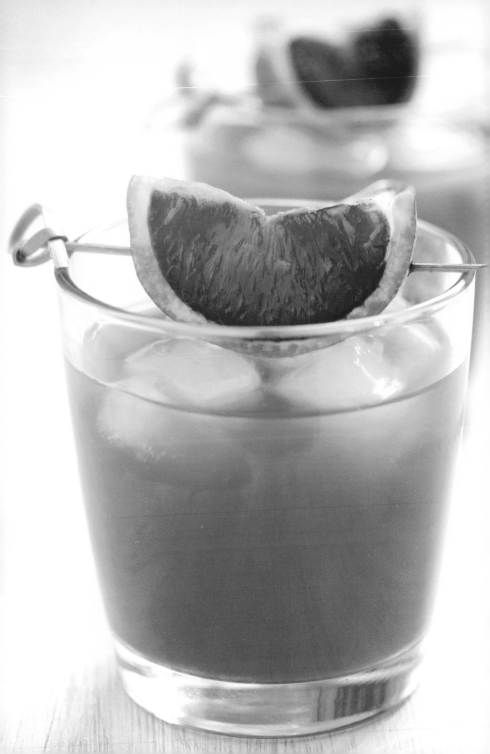

STRAWBERRY FIELDS JUICE

Fresh strawberry juice? You bet! This one is blended with cucumber, orange, and carrots for a delicious blend of fruits and veggies.

---

 2 cups strawberries, stems removed

 ½ cucumber

 1 blood orange, peeled and sectioned

 2 carrots

Combine all ingredients in a juicer. Pour juice into a glass or over ice, garnish with a skewered section of blood orange if you'd like, and drink immediately.

Bonus Recipe

STRAWBERRY FIELDS SMOOTHIE

 Leave out the cucumber and carrot. Blend your fresh strawberry-orange juice with ¾ cup plain Greek yogurt and ice cubes to taste.

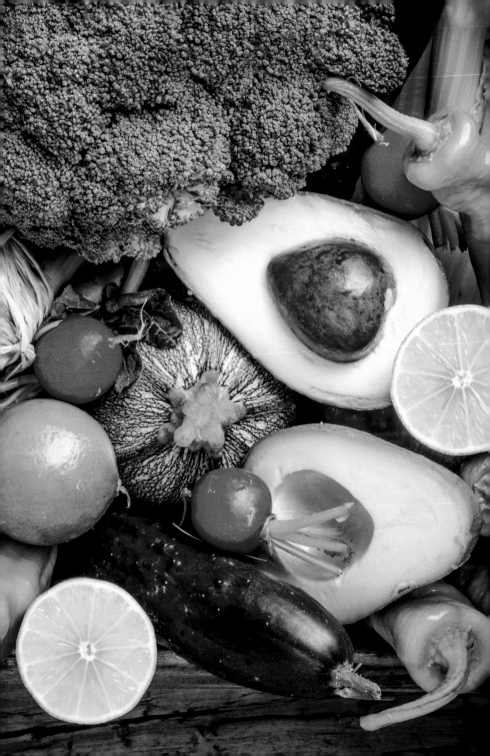

VEGETABLE JUICE BLENDS

*If you're falling short on your daily intake
of fresh vegetables, these juice blends are for you!*
Some of these juices have a half-dozen different veggie
varieties in them. How's that for drinking the rainbow?
Freshly pressed juice makes it easy to get a plethora
of vitamins and minerals in your diet.

The majority of these vegetable juice blends tend
to have an earthy, sometimes bitter flavor. You might love
how these different vegetable tastes meld together,
but if they're too strong for you, try diluting the juice
with water or mellowing out the flavor by juicing an apple,
pear, or cucumber along with the other ingredients.
There's no wrong way to make juice. In fact, the only
right way to make it is when you love the taste.
Don't be afraid to experiment.

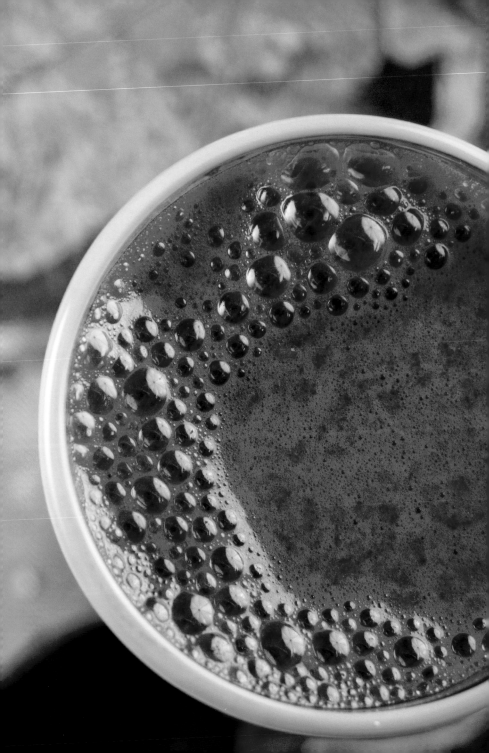

V3 JUICE

Made with just three different vegetables, this simple juice comes together in a matter of minutes and, boy, does it pack a nutritional punch. Packed with vitamin A, C, folate, fiber, and whole slew of antioxidants, this juice will make you feel a tad bit healthier starting with the very first sip.

 2 beets

 5 carrots

 1 cucumber

Combine all ingredients in a juicer. Pour juice into a glass or over ice and drink immediately.

Bonus Recipe

POWER PUNCH
Juice 2 beets, 3 carrots, 1 cucumber, 2 celery stalks, and ½ lemon, peeled and segmented.

"Eat food. Not too much. Mostly plants."

— MICHAEL POLLAN

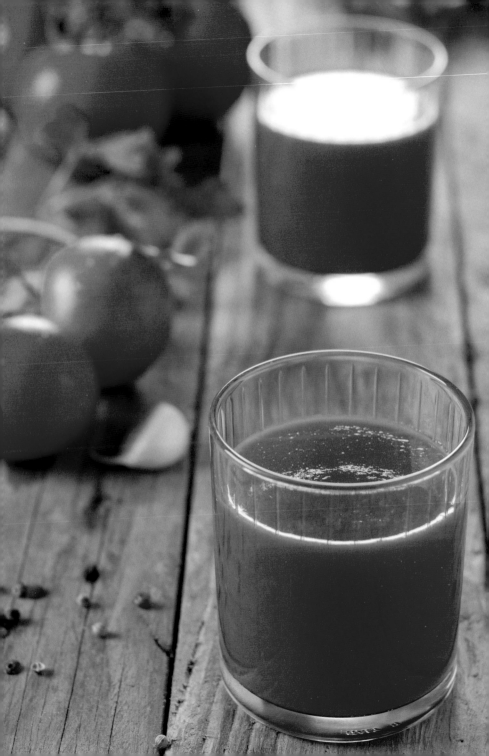

VERY VEGGIE JUICE

Start your day on the right foot with this winning combination of vegetables. You'll get a whole slew of nutrients in each sip.

 3 medium tomatoes

 2 carrots

 2 celery stalks

 ½ lemon

 1 clove of garlic, peeled

 1 piece of horseradish to taste *optional*

 Sea salt to taste *optional*

Combine all ingredients in a juicer. Pour juice into a glass or over ice and drink immediately.

Bonus Recipe

SPICY VEGGIE JUICE

 For an extra-spicy vegetable juice, add ½ jalapeño pepper before juicing.

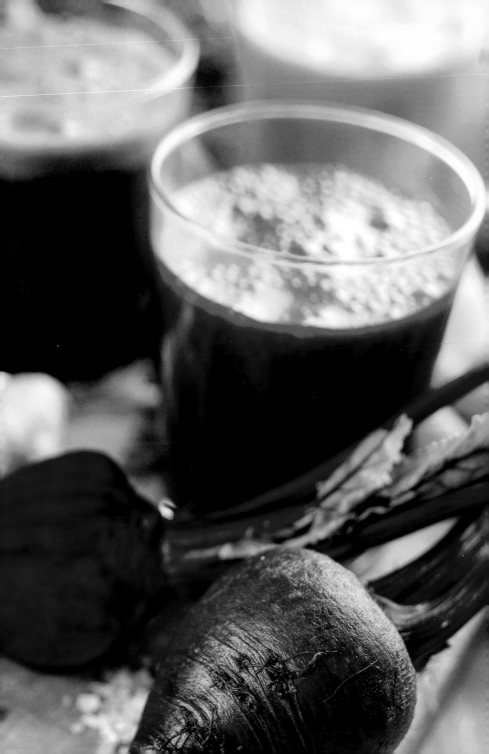

BEETLE JUICE

You'll love how you feel after drinking it this beet-based juice, loaded with essential vitamins and nutrients.

---

 4 ounces Swiss chard or spinach

 1 apple

 2 beets

 2 celery stalks

 ½ lemon *optional*

 Freshly ground pepper to taste *optional*

Put ingredients into a juicer, alternating greens with chunked fruits and veggies. Pour into a glass and drink immediately.

Bonus Recipe

 ## FEISTY BEETLE JUICE
Add a generous amount of fresh ginger root before juicing.

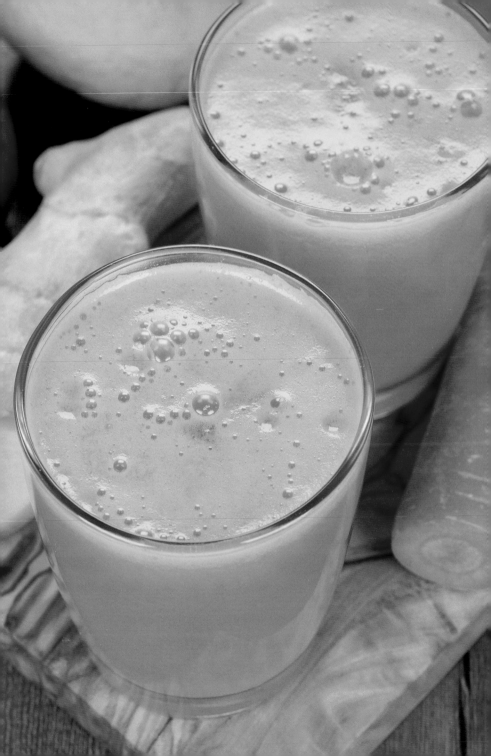

CARROT WITH A KICK

This isn't your regular glass of carrot juice! Thanks to apple, lemon, and ginger, this one has a little sweet, a little sour, and a whole lot of zip.

 6–8 carrots

 1 apple

 ½ lemon

 Fresh ginger root to taste

Combine all ingredients in a juicer. Pour juice into a glass or over ice and drink immediately.

Bonus Recipe

CARROT-CLEMENTINE JUICE
Replace the apple with a clementine, peeled and segmented.

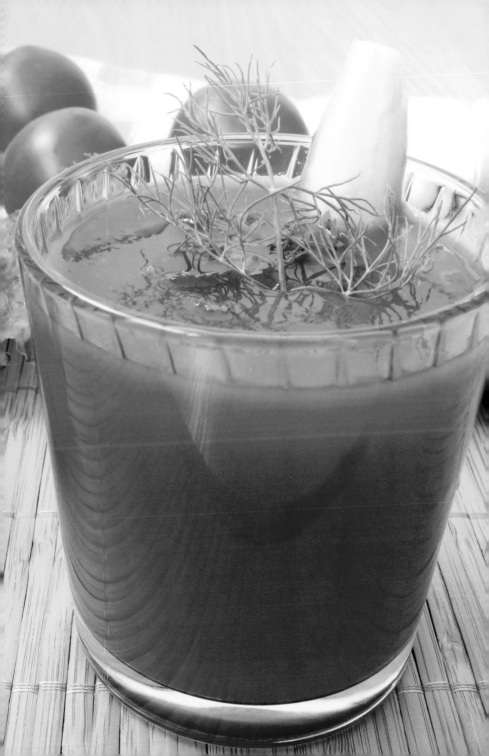

TOMATO-DILL JUICE

Fresh dill complements tomato so well in this juice. Add a touch of sea salt and freshly ground pepper for a savory juice full of flavor.

---

 4 tomatoes

 ½ cucumber

 1 bunch of dill

 Sea salt to taste

 Pepper to taste

Combine all ingredients in a juicer. Pour juice into a glass or over ice. Garnish with a lemon wedge, piece of dill, or celery sticks, and drink immediately.

Bonus Recipe

 ## MARY'S MOCKTAIL
Take some inspiration from the classic Bloody Mary cocktail and add three dashes of hot sauce.

Who knew? Chew fresh dill to help alleviate halitosis (bad breath)!

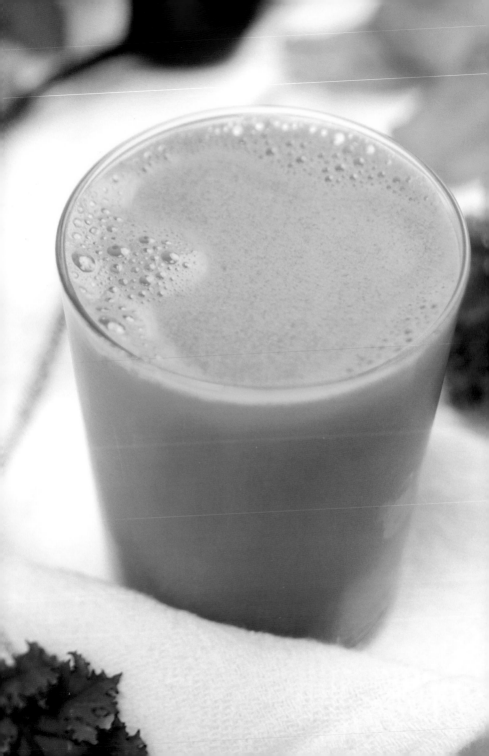

GOLDEN BEET-CITRUS JUICE

Golden beets tend to have a mellow and earthy taste, so when combined with bold citrus, you'll be pleasantly surprised with how greatly these flavors are enhanced. And, of course, you'll love the eye-catching colors in this juice!

---

 2 small golden beets or one large

 4 carrots

 1 orange, peeled and sectioned

 ½ apple

 Fresh ginger root to taste *optional*

Combine all ingredients in a juicer. Pour juice into a glass or over ice and drink immediately.

Bonus Recipe

BEET-RED CITRUS JUICE
Use red beets instead of golden ones for a deeper flavor and color.

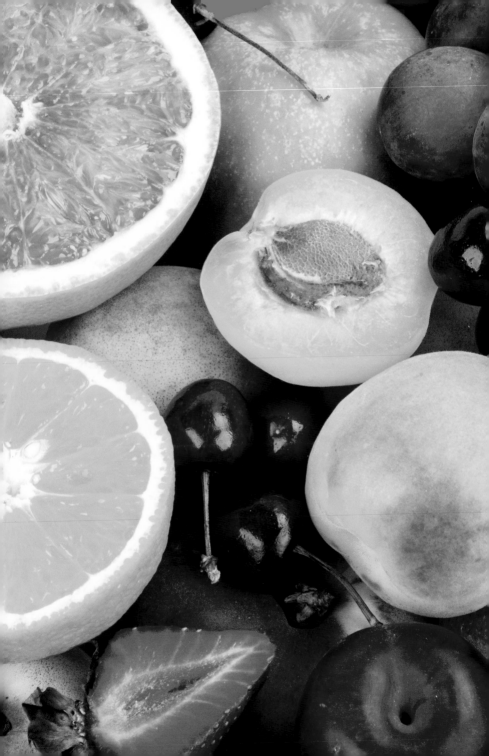

ENERGIZING SMOOTHIES AND JUICES

Are you dragging today? Lacking focus? Feel like taking a nap? Instead of reaching for a cup of coffee or brownie—both of which give you a temporary jolt of energy—try one of these energy-boosting juices. Drinking caffeine or eating a sweet treat may help you feel better quickly, but it's only temporary. The caffeine or sugar high usually wears off in an hour or so, which puts you right back where you started (and possibly feeling worse than before).

The recipes in this chapter are a natural remedy to help combat that sluggish feeling. They're filled with ingredients that will naturally boost your energy and get you going. Drink them first thing in the morning or in the afternoon to prevent that post-lunch slump.

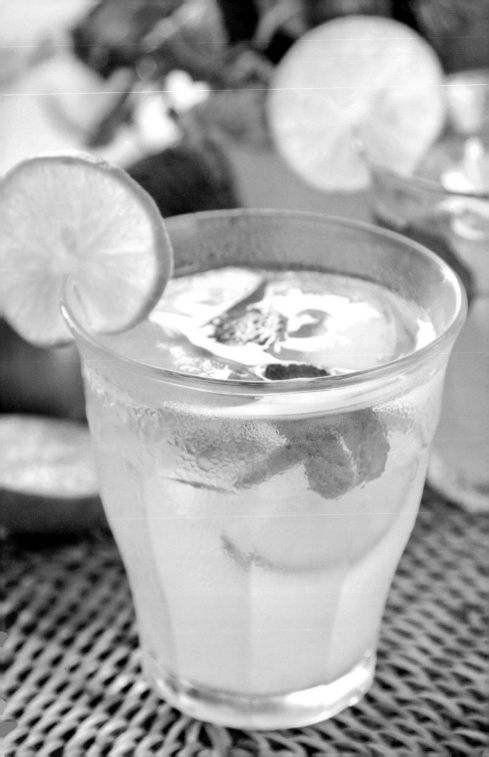

COCONUT-LIME JUICE

Coconut water is incredibly hydrating, which will give you an instant boost if you're feeling a little parched. Juiced with fresh lime, apple, and spinach, it'll provide your body with a whole host of feel-good nutrients.

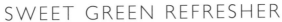

 1 lime, peeled and segmented

 ½ apple

 1 cup coconut water

Put fruits into the juicer. Combine with the coconut water, pour into a glass, and drink immediately.

Bonus Recipe

 ## SWEET GREEN REFRESHER
For an extra nutrition boost, add a handful of spinach to the ingredients for juicing.

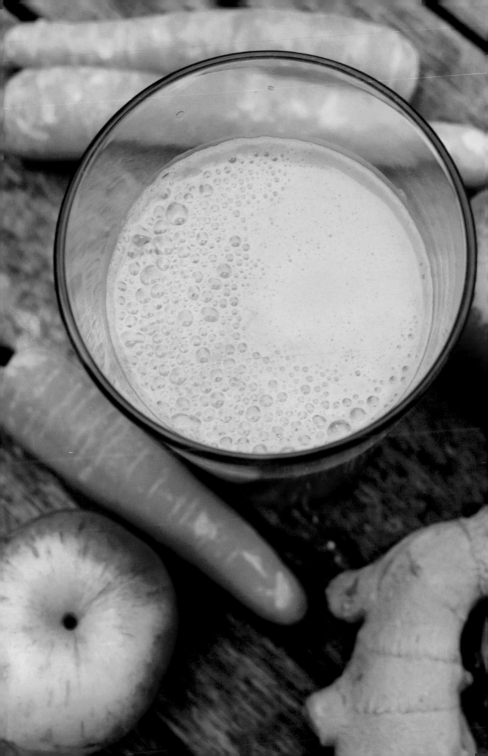

CARROT-GINGER-APPLE JUICE

This colorful, zesty mixture of carrot, apple, and fresh ginger will wake up your senses and give you an instant, natural lift. Drink this juice whenever you feel the need to be revived.

 5–6 carrots

 2 apples

 Fresh ginger to taste

Combine all ingredients in a juicer. Pour juice into a glass or over ice and drink immediately.

Bonus Recipe

CARROT-GINGER-GRAPEFRUIT JUICE
Omit apples and add one pink grapefruit.

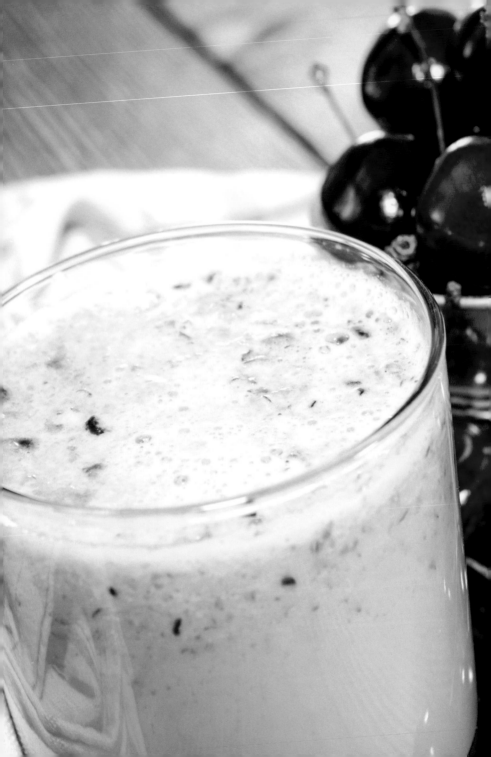

CHERRY-PINEAPPLE REFRESHER

Drinking a brightly-colored, nutrient-rich glass of juice is a great way to instantly give you a lift, and this juice does just that. Even your taste buds will be wide awake.

 1 Granny Smith apple

 2 cups pineapple, cut into chunks

 1 cup pitted cherries

 ½ lemon *optional*

 8–10 mint leaves

Combine all ingredients in a juicer. Pour juice into a glass or over ice and drink immediately.

Bonus Recipe

  ## CHERRY-PINEAPPLE JUICE
Leave out the apple and lemon and instead juice 1 cup of watermelon or cantaloupe. If you use watermelon, be sure to remove any seeds.

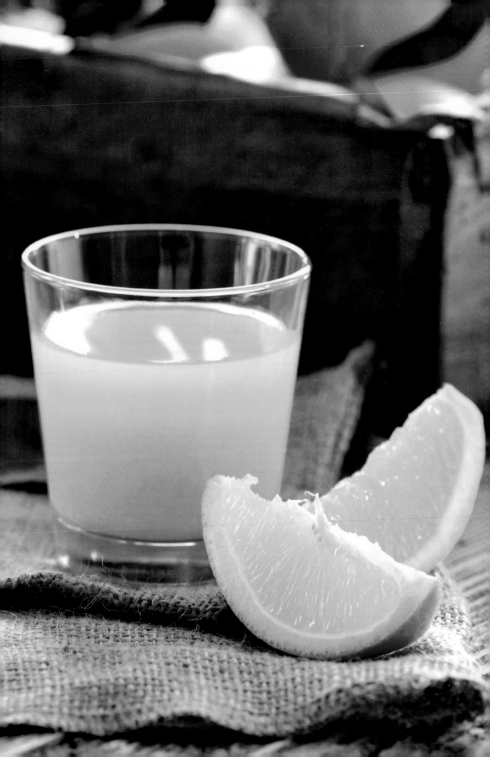

SUNSHINE CITRUS JUICE

When you're feeling lethargic and low on energy, skip the energy drink and reach for this sweet citrus blend. Instead of a quick boost that will leave you crashing sooner than later, this juice will give you long-lasting energy.

---

 2 oranges, peeled and sectioned

 2 apples

 I sweet potato

Combine all ingredients in a juice. Pour juice into a glass or over ice and drink immediately.

Bonus Recipe

SUNSET CREAMSICLE

 For a milky alternative, add ¼ cup to ½ cup of almond milk after juicing the other ingredients. Stir and enjoy.

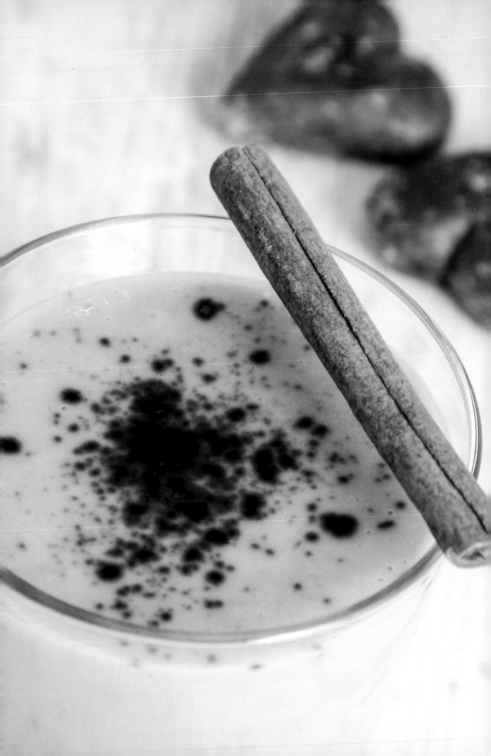

JAVA JOLT SMOOTHIE

Need a little pick-me-up? Look no further! This smoothie will give you the energy you need to help you sail through your day.

 I frozen banana

 2 tbsp almond butter

 I cup almond milk

 I ounce espresso

 I tsp honey (or agave nectar)

 ½ tsp vanilla extract

 ½ tsp cinnamon

4–5 ice cubes

Combine ingredients in a blender until smooth. Pour into a glass, garnish with a cinnamon stick if desired, and enjoy immediately.

Bonus Recipe

 ## CHOCOLATE JAVA SMOOTHIE
Add 2 tbsp of carob or dark chocolate chips.

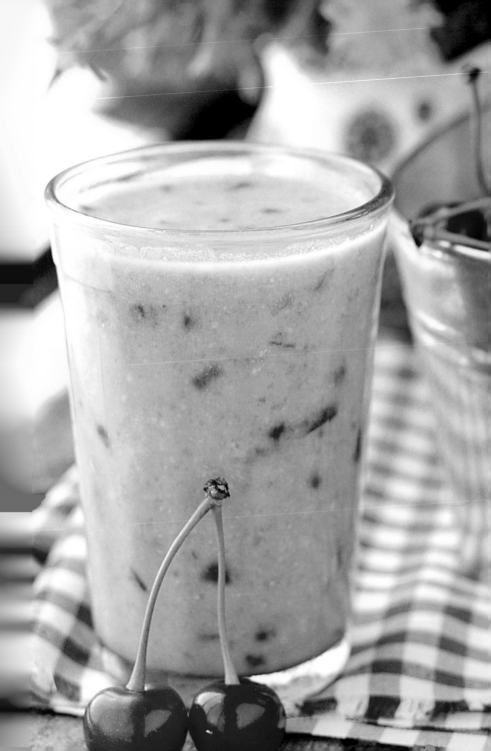

CHERRY-VANILLA SMOOTHIE

Sweet and creamy, you'll love enjoying cherries this way. A serving of yogurt adds creaminess and flavor along with some healthy fats and protein to keep you satisfied.

I cup frozen pitted cherries

6 ounces yogurt (preferably vanilla-flavored)

½ cup vanilla almond milk

½ tsp vanilla extract

Combine ingredients in a blender until smooth. Pour into a glass and enjoy immediately.

Bonus Recipe

CHERRY CRUMBLE SMOOTHIE
For an even thicker and more satisfying smoothie, add ¼ cup of rolled oats along with an additional ½ cup of almond milk before blending.

CHOOSING A JUICER

Electric juicers come in two main types: masticating (also known as cold press because they don't produce heat when they extract the juice) and centrifugal.

A masticating juicer works by smashing and crushing fruits and vegetables and then squeezing them through a fine, stainless steel strainer to produce juice. This type of juicer tends to be quieter and extracts more juice and nutrients because it generates less heat and friction. But masticating juicers also tend to be bulkier and more expensive than centrifugal juicers.

A centrifugal juicer has sharp, fast-spinning metal blades that shred the fruits and vegetables and then, using centrifugal force, separate the juice from the pulp, which are then separated into different containers. Some centrifugal juicers have an automatic pulp ejector that sends the pulp into a side container once the juice has been extracted, which makes cleanup easier and faster. Other centrifugal juicers have an extra-wide mouth that allows you to feed larger pieces of fruit and vegetables into the machine, which reduces the time spent cutting up produce to be juiced.

In the end, it's up to you which kind of juicer fits into your lifestyle and budget. If you're not too picky about getting the most nutrients or don't have a lot of money to spend, the centrifugal juicer might be for you. However, if you want to pack the most nutrients as possible into your body and don't mind spending a few extra bucks, go for the masticating (cold press) juicer.

No matter what you decide, consider the ease of use of the juicer you choose. The easier it is to use—and clean!—your juicer, the more often you'll use it.

INDEX

ABOUT CIDER MILL PRESS
BOOK PUBLISHERS

Good ideas ripen with time. From seed to harvest, Cider Mill Press brings fine reading, information, and entertainment together between the covers of its creatively crafted books. Our Cider Mill bears fruit twice a year, publishing a new crop of titles each spring and fall.

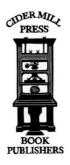

Visit us on the Web at
www.cidermillpress.com
or write to us at
12 Spring Street
PO Box 454
Kennebunkport, Maine 04046